Lovers'
massage

Lovers'
massage
Soothing Touch for Two

Darrin Zeer
Illustrations by Amy Saidens

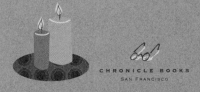

CHRONICLE BOOKS
SAN FRANCISCO

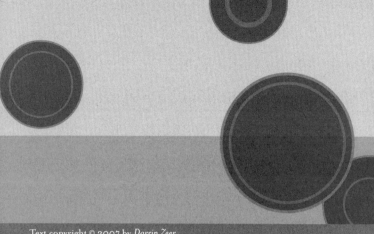

Library of Congress Cataloging-in-Publication
Data available.

ISBN-10: 0-8118-4944-9
ISBN-13: 978-0-8118-4944-9

Manufactured in China.

Design by Tana Martin

Distributed in Canada by Raincoast Books
9050 Shaughnessy Street
Vancouver, British Columbia V6P 6E5

10 9 8 7 6 5 4 3 2 1

Chronicle Books LLC
680 Second Street
San Francisco, California 94107
www.chroniclebooks.com

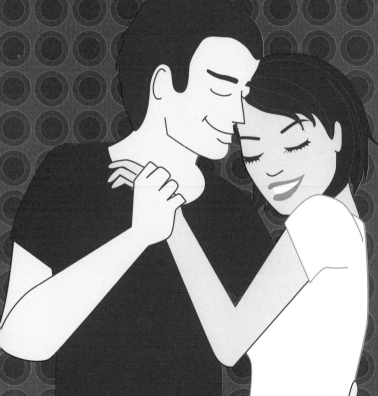

Contents

Quickie Help Guide

Learn the Fabulous Five Massages!

Take a Mini Romantic Getaway!

Introduction

*Give your partner a Lovers' Massage,
it's a fabulous way to say "I love you"!*

After a long day at work, the last thing we usually want to do is "give" to our partner. We're just too pooped. We want only to veg out in front of the TV. So, the challenge is, how can we find the time or the energy to take care of our own needs and at the same time nurture and stay connected with our partner?

Lovers' Massage is the perfect activity for couples desiring to spend time together. When you practice massage and stretching with your partner, you function beautifully as your own stress-management team. The physical contact between the two of you melts away your stress and reignites your passion. A profound connection occurs as you enjoy touch together. This special time with your partner helps make for a healthier, happier relationship. What could be more efficient than a bodywork program that is easy to do, gives both of you peace of mind, rejuvenates your bodies, and creates more love and intimacy?

Lovers' Massage is a special blend of ancient massage and stretching techniques that originate from the Far East. For thousands of years throughout Asia, people have been practicing Shiatsu, Thai Yoga Massage, and many other advanced bodywork traditions. This book borrows from these age-old practices and has especially adapted them for couples. Learn a whole new way to give a deep, nurturing massage that usually doesn't require you to lift a finger. Rest your tired hands, and let the rest of your body do the

work for you. You will master how to massage with your feet, knees, elbows, and entire body.

This book is broken up into five parts—rejuvenating, relaxing, reconnecting, reviving, and romantic—an exotic blend of more than fifty massage techniques. You don't have to be strong, and you don't have to be experienced; you just have to be willing to give and receive. Forget all your insecurities about giving a good massage. By combining both massage and stretching, you will hit the right spot every time, and your partner will be in bliss. I guarantee it!

During and after a Lovers' Massage session, you'll feel an irresistible desire to hug and cuddle with your partner. An intimate, caring space is created that you can return to at any time. Whether you have just a minute in the morning, some time in front of the TV, or an entire romantic weekend, try one or many of these Lovers' Massage techniques, and you'll relaxingly experience amazing results. Don't miss out on the "Fabulous Five Massages" and "Mini Romantic Getaway" sections at the end of each of the chapters. If you are short on time and need a fast fix, try the "Quickie Help Guide" in front, on page 7.

Enjoy deep relaxation and profound intimacy with your partner!

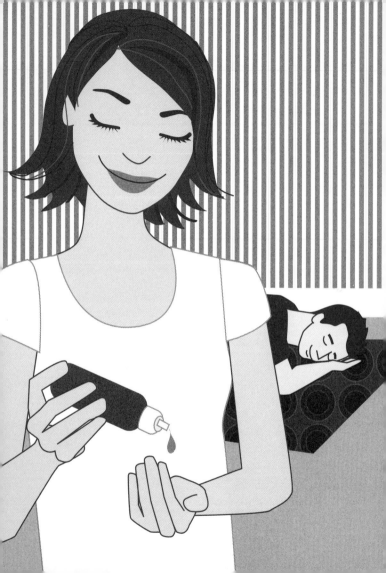

Partner Preparation

Before you give a massage session, it's helpful to spend a few moments to calm and prepare yourself. Take a few long, deep breaths, and focus on relaxing your body. Please review these points for the receiver and giver.

Instructions for Receiving

•••• Trust the giver to take good care of your body. Tell the giver if you want more or less massage pressure.

•••• Don't hesitate to be vocal; tell your partner when it feels good. Don't hold back your compliments.

•••• Let your entire body relax as you get your massage.

•••• Remember to take long, deep breaths!

•••• When you feel tightness in your body, focus on breathing and letting go of the tension.

Instructions for Giving

•••• Massage the receiver's body with love and care.

•••• Don't forget to ask the receiver if he or she is feeling good and how he or she likes the massage pressure throughout the session.

•••• Make sure your body is always comfortably positioned. Remember to enjoy yourself, and don't work hard.

•••• Be spontaneous and creative! Feel free to experiment and create your own special massage moves.

•••• Have some massage oil or lotion close by.

Creating Your Couple's Sanctuary

····· For best results, practice Lovers' Massage on a large futon or a comforter on the floor. You can also do this series on your bed, but skip the standing-massage techniques.

- Shower and freshen up: wear loose, comfortable clothing that feels good to stretch in!

- Use mints for fresh breath, and have drinking water available.

- Take breaks, and feed each other tasty snacks like pieces of fruit or chocolate. Present your snacks on a fancy tray.

- Turn all the phones off; find a quiet, private space; and limit all distractions.

- Play music to set an intimate mood. Have a selection of your favorite love songs that you both enjoy.

- Dim the lights, and light some candles.

- Keep pillows and blankets handy. Make sure neither of you gets chilly.

- Use natural water-based massage-oil products that won't stain clothes or bedding. Choose a scent that you know your partner loves.

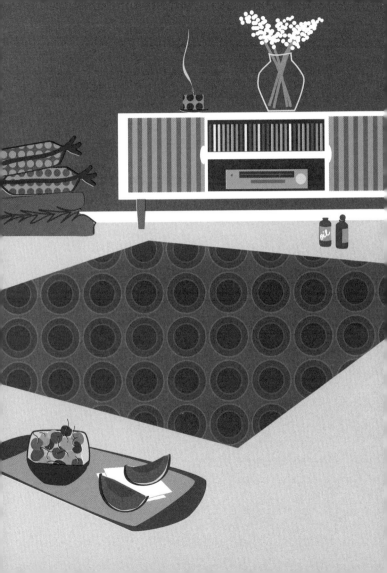

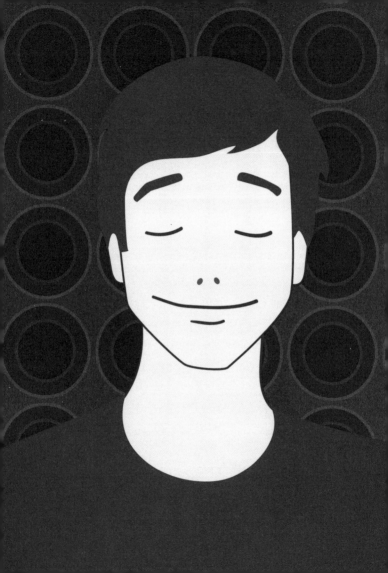

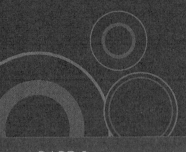

PART 1:
Rejuvenating Partner Massage
Stimulating Leg Series

This massage series will stimulate the energy flow through the feet and legs, and is both energizing and relaxing.

Nice Legs
Sole Squeeze

- Your partner lies faceup, with her feet two feet apart.
- Put a pillow under her head if she likes.
- Kneel at her feet, sitting on your knees between her legs.
- Rest your hands on her feet, and sit motionless for a few deep breaths together.
- Slowly rock your body forward and back, squeezing your partner's feet on each backward rocking motion.
- Use your body weight as leverage to apply deeper pressure.
- Squeeze your hands around her feet, from toes to heels and back again.
- Ask her how she likes the pressure.
- Push her feet downward with your hands, and hold for a few breaths.
- Pound lightly the soles of her feet with loose fists.
- Take hold of her ankles, lean back, and pull her legs.

Leg Squeeze

- Massage with your thumbs along the inside of her legs to the top of her thighs and then back down to the feet.
- Remember to maintain a gentle, slow rhythm to help her relax.
- Take long, deep breaths together.

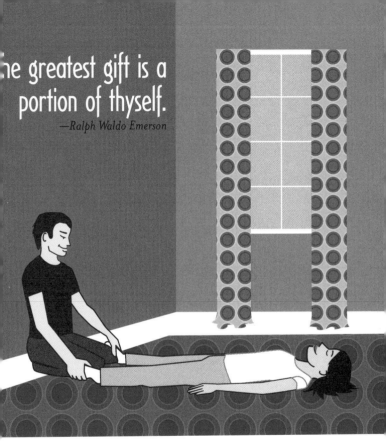

The greatest gift is a portion of thyself.
—*Ralph Waldo Emerson*

Healing Benefits: *Stimulates energy flow and increases flexibility in the leg and feet joints.*

Romantic Stroll

Single Leg Walk

- Your partner lies faceup, with his feet two feet apart.

- Sit down between his feet, with your legs stretched out in front of you.

- Gently bend his left knee up using your right foot.

- Firmly grip both of his ankles for extra leverage.

- Apply pressure with your right foot on his left thigh, and hold.

- Lean back and pull his ankles to increase your foot pressure.

- Walk your foot slowly up and down his thigh region and gently apply pressure.

- Ask him if he wants more or less foot pressure.

- Try not to pinch the skin on his leg while you walk with your foot.

Double Leg Walk

- Keep a firm grip on his ankles, and walk both your feet on his left thigh.

- Walk all over his thigh firmly.

- Ask him how he likes the pressure.

- Enjoy yourself, and be creative with this technique.

- Take deep, relaxing breaths together.

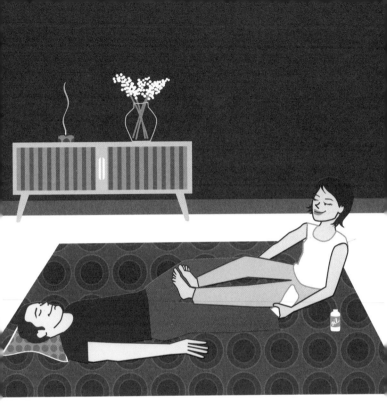

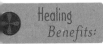

Relieves leg and lower-back tightness.

Thigh Master

- Brace your feet on her inner left thigh, tucked in snugly behind her knee.

- Bend her left lower leg across both your shins.

- Stretch your body forward, and use your hands to grasp the front surface of her thigh.

- Alternately massage and pull with both your hands along the length of her upper thigh.

- Enjoy a good forward stretch while you massage her.

Shake a Leg

- Walk your right foot on her left thigh and your left foot on her right thigh at the same time.

- Hold both her ankles firmly for extra leverage.

- Lean back, and rock her legs back and forth and side to side.

- Ask her how the foot pressure feels.

- Relax, and have some fun experimenting with this technique.

Repeat both series on her other leg.

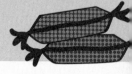

Healing Benefits: *Loosens tightness in the hamstrings, thighs, and hips.*

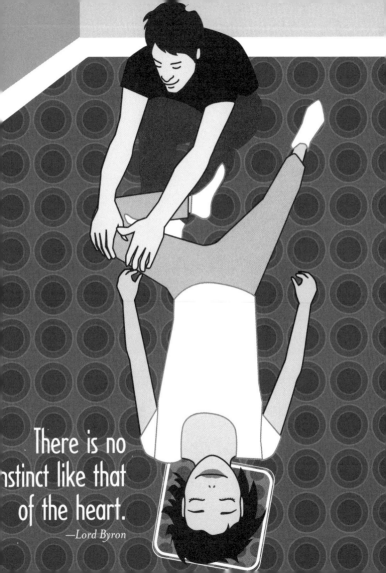

There is no
instinct like that
of the heart.
—*Lord Byron*

Leg Hugs
Calf Squeeze

- Your partner lies faceup.

- Kneel in front of his left leg.

- Bend his left leg, and lock his left foot between your knees.

- Interlace your fingers together behind his calf.

- Rock forward and back, massaging his calf with your interlaced hands.

- Lean back as far as you can, so he will get a nice hip stretch.

- This will increase the pressure on the calf as well as extend and open the hip.

Repeat on his other leg.

Thigh Squeeze

- Interlace your fingers, and place them across the top of his thigh just above his knee.

- Squeeze firmly with your palms, and massage the full length of his thigh.

- Lean your upper body forward, and rest your chest on his knee.

- Remind him to take deep, relaxing breaths.

- Say something simple to your partner like, "I love having you in my life."

Repeat on his other leg.

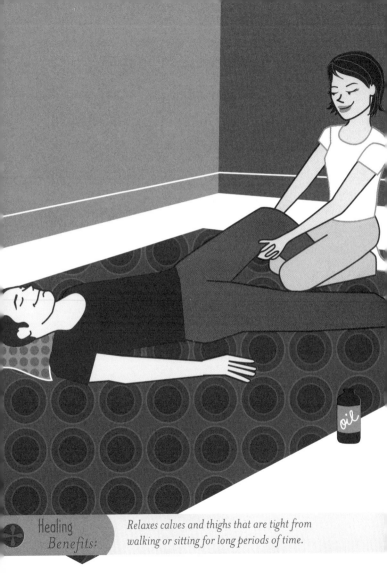

Healing Benefits: *Relaxes calves and thighs that are tight from walking or sitting for long periods of time.*

Leg Wrestling
Kneeing Thigh

- Your partner lies faceup.
- Squat down in front of his legs.
- Lift and bend his left knee toward his chest.
- Hold his left ankle and knee with your hands, and brace your right foot for balance.
- Press your right knee into the back side of his left thigh.
- Pull his left foot to apply more knee pressure.

Advanced move: bend both of his legs, rest his ankles on your shoulders, and gently lower both your knees down onto the back sides of his thighs.

Forearm Squeeze

- Kneel to the outside of his left leg.
- Lift and bend his left knee toward his chest.
- Tuck your right forearm tightly in behind his left knee.
- Press his ankle gently downward to create a squeeze on his calf and thigh.
- Ask him how he likes the pressure.
- Make sure you both are taking long, deep breaths together.

Advanced move: bend both of his legs, and place both of your forearms in between the calves and back sides of his thighs. Lean forward, and use your upper body for leverage.

Repeat both series on his other leg.

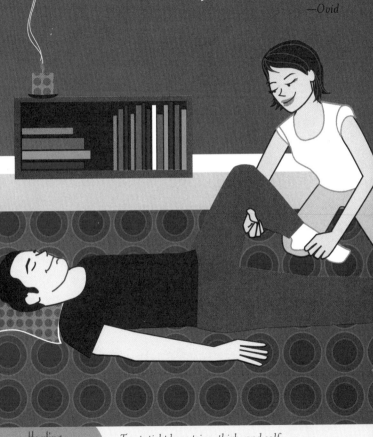

Fortune and love favor the brave.

—*Ovid*

Healing Benefits: *Treats tight hamstring, thigh, and calf muscles and stimulates blood flow.*

Intimate Partner Pleasure

Happy Hip Twist

- Your partner lies faceup, with her feet two feet apart.

- Kneel between her legs.

- Bend her legs up, and push her knees to her chest.

- Lower both of her knees slowly to her left side.

- Gently massage her right hip and buttocks with your palms, knuckles, and forearms.

- Caringly remind her to relax; feel the rhythm of love between you.

- Take five or more deep breaths together.

- Slowly lift her legs back up, and repeat this series on her other side.

Buddy Butterfly Opening

- Rest the soles of her feet on top of your crossed legs on either side of your belly.

- Slowly let her knees drop out in opposite directions; your bent legs will act as a support for her legs.

- Gently massage her inner thighs and calves with your hands and forearms.

- Take five or more deep breaths together.

- Ask her if she would like her legs stretched apart farther.

- Very slowly and gently raise her knees back together.

Gratitude is the heart's memory.
—French proverb

Healing Benefits: Opens up the hip, groin, and lower-back region.

Fabulous Five Massages

Love Seat

Sit cross-legged closely together, and hug.

Use this time to connect with your hearts.

Heart to heart!

You can loosely wrap your legs around each other.

Rest your head on your partner's shoulder.

Take five or more deep breaths together, and relax.

Spend time massaging your partner's back.

Show how much you care through your touch.

Rub the muscles along each side of the spine, especially around the shoulder blades.

Ask your partner how the pressure feels and which areas need attention.

Focus on letting your bodies melt into each other.

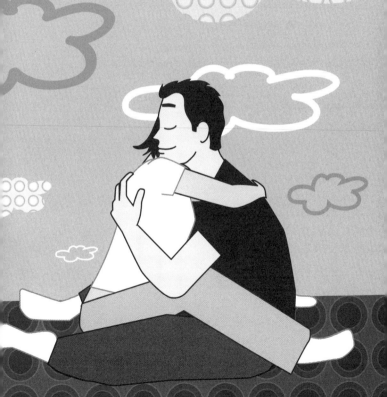

At the touch of love everyone becomes a poet.
—*Plato*

· Mini Romantic Getaway ·
Footbath Bliss

· · · · · · When your partner gets home from a long day at work, offer him or her a luxurious footbath.

· · · · · · Prepare a warm bowl in which to soak your partner's feet.

· · · · · · Use soap or essential oils or both.

· · · · · · Have your partner sit back and close his or her eyes.

· · · · · · Soak your partner's feet in the warm water, and gently caress each foot.

· · · · · · Use firm finger pressure on the sole of each foot.

· · · · · · Wrap your partner's feet in a soft towel, and dry each foot.

· · · · · · Give each foot some soft, sweet kisses as an expression of your love.

· · · · · · If it feels right, check in with your partner and ask about his or her day.

· · · · · · Listen closely and with care!

Being deeply loved by someone gives you strength; loving someone deeply gives you courage.

—Lao Tzu

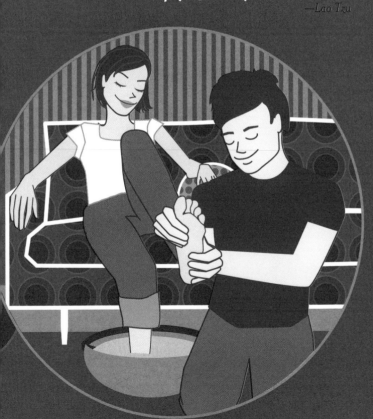

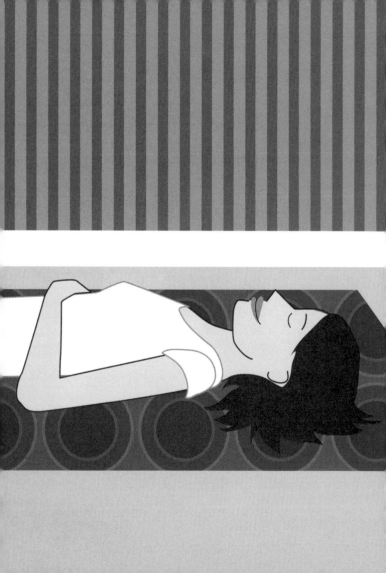

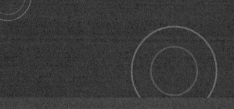

PART 2:
Relaxing Partner Massage
Stress-Relieving Upper-Body Series

This massage series will stimulate the energy flow
in the upper back and is very stress-relieving.

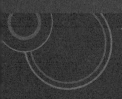

Stretching Sandwich
Head to Knee

- Your partner lies faceup.

- Lift his legs until they are straight up in front of your legs and belly.

- Lean forward, and firmly grip each other's forearms or wrists.

- Lean back, and pull his upper body upward.

- He should feel a stretch in his back.

- Hold the position for as long as possible, and then gently lower him.

- Repeat this series twice, and maintain a slow, steady rhythm throughout.

Head to Crossed Leg

- Keep holding his legs up.

- Bend his knees outward, crossing his ankles in front of your knees.

- Adjust his position so that the sides of both of his ankles are resting against your shins.

- Now, firmly grip each other's forearms or wrists, and raise his upper body toward you once more.

- Hold for as long as comfortable, release, and repeat this series twice.

- Make sure you both breathe and relax during these stretches.

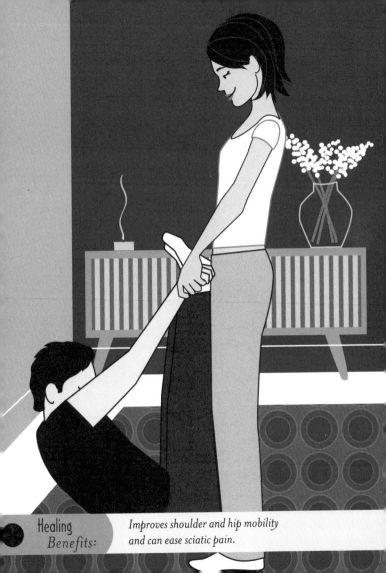

Healing Benefits: *Improves shoulder and hip mobility and can ease sciatic pain.*

Passion Pretzel

••••• *This is an intense stretch and is not for everyone.*

- Your partner lies faceup.

- Stand at her feet, and lift her legs straight up in the air.

- Step between her legs to where you can easily position your feet under her armpits.

- Bend your knees slightly, and, reaching behind, slowly pull her legs around the outsides of your legs.

- Bring the soles of her feet together in front of you and slightly downward.

- Be very gentle, and ask her how the stretch feels.

- Stretch her feet toward her head to raise her buttocks up off the ground.

- Hold this stretch for five deep breaths.

- Release her from this stretch slowly, and relax.

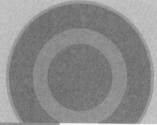

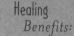

Healing *Benefits:* Aids mobility of the hip joints and eases lower back pain.

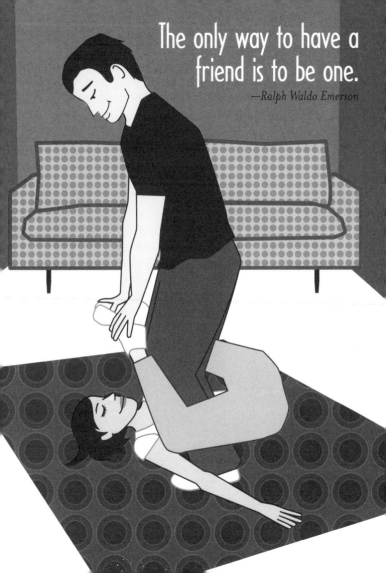

The only way to have a
friend is to be one.
—*Ralph Waldo Emerson*

Belly Dance
Belly Circles

- Your partner lies faceup.

- Kneel by his left side, near his belly, and place your hands on his belly.

- Invite him to take five deep breaths.

- Press with your palms and fingers, and make slow clockwise circles around his belly.

- Rock your body forward slowly, moving your hands rhythmically.

- Use your hands to tune into your partner's breathing.

Belly Press

- Cover his navel with your palms.

- Have him lift his belly up against the pressure of your hands as he breathes in.

- Gently press down on his belly to offer gentle resistance.

- Apply more pressure with your palms, gradually, each time he exhales.

- Invite him to take five deep, long breaths.

Healing Benefits: *Aids digestion and relieves constipation and premenstrual discomfort.*

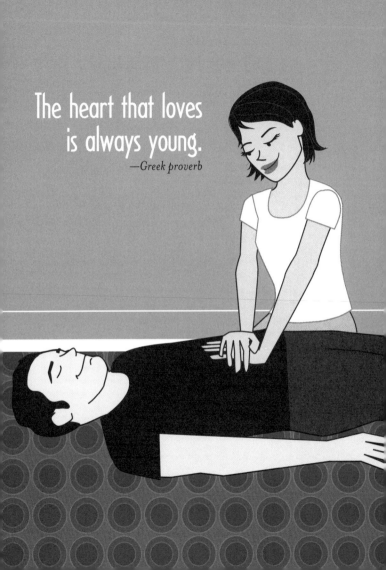

The heart that loves
is always young.
—*Greek proverb*

Head Games
Head Heaven

- Your partner lies faceup.
- Sit cross-legged at her head.
- Place one hand underneath her head, making sure not to pull her hair, and one hand on her forehead.
- Cradle her head, relax, and take five deep breaths together, motionless.
- You may want to lubricate your hands with a few drops of massage oil or lotion.
- Then, slide one hand after the other under her neck, and pull gently toward you to create a soothing traction for her spine.
- Repeat several times in a slow, rhythmic motion.
- Whisper sweet nothings into her ear.

Neck and Scalp Serenity

- Lift her head up, and slide her head to the right side.
- It helps to lubricate your hands with a few drops of massage oil or lotion.
- Brace her head with your right hand.
- Gently massage her neck between the ear and shoulder with the knuckles from your left hand.
- Simultaneously massage her scalp with your right hand.
- Next, roll her head over onto the right temple.
- Press along the full length of the neck muscles with your left thumb.
- Ask her if she wants more or less pressure.
  Repeat this series on the other side.

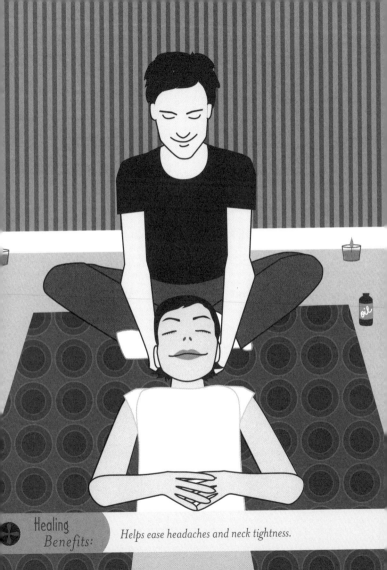

Healing
Benefits: *Helps ease headaches and neck tightness.*

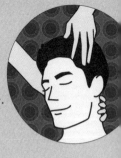

Neck Figure Eights

- Brace your hands underneath his head, making sure not to pull his hair.

- Slowly rotate his head in circles, turning his head in a figure-eight motion.

- Move his head from side to side and up and down.

- Go slow, relax, and breathe together.

- Next, lift his head straight up, moving his chin to his chest.

- Brace his head up with your crossed hands.

- Lean forward, using your body weight for extra leverage.

- Hold for a few deep breaths, and ask if he wants more or less of a stretch.

Happy Head

- Sit behind his head, and, bending your knees, place your feet on his shoulders.

- Cradle each side of his head with your hands.

- Gently hold the weight of his head by your fingertips.

- Create traction by pushing the soles of your feet on his shoulders.

- Ask him how it feels, relax, and breathe!

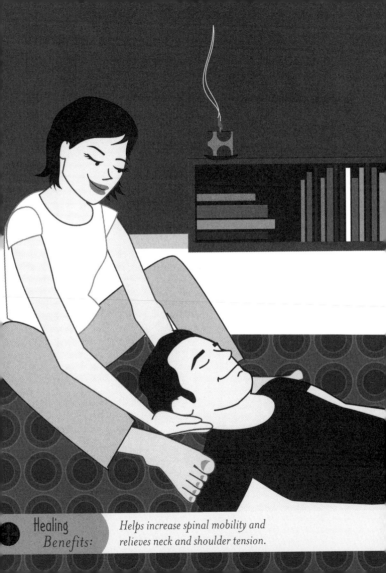

Healing Benefits: *Helps increase spinal mobility and relieves neck and shoulder tension.*

fulfilling facial

- Your partner lies faceup.

- Sit cross-legged above her head, and rest her head on your ankles. You can use a pillow for her head to rest on.

- Lubricate your hands with a few drops of massage oil or lotion.

- Place your thumbs on the center of her forehead just above the brow.

- Firmly slide your thumbs outward toward her temples.

- Repeat this technique all over the forehead.

- Circle your thumbs or fingers gently around the temples several times.

- Rest your hands on the sides of her head, and make small circles with your thumbs from the inner to outer edge of her eyebrows.

- Rub your fingertips in a circular motion on her cheekbones and jaw.

- Squeeze the outside edge of her ears, using your thumbs and fingertips.

- Softly caress your fingers over her face, and feel the love you have for her.

- To complete, rub your hands together quickly to create heat, and place your hands gently over her eyes and face.

- Hold motionless for a few moments.

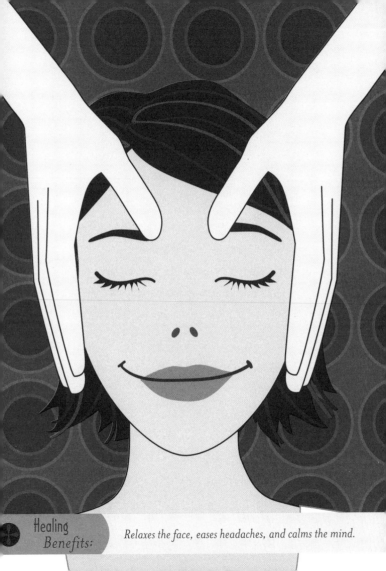

Relaxes the face, eases headaches, and calms the mind.

Fabulous Five Massages

Heavenly Pose

- Sit on the ground, legs outstretched.

- Help your partner sit in front of you but facing away, with legs also outstretched.

- Place some pillows behind your back for support, and lie down backward.

- Gently ease your partner's body back, with his or her head resting on your belly or chest.

- Guide your partner to completely relax.

- You may need a small pillow to cushion your partner's head.

- Rest both of your hands on your partner's shoulders.

- If you can reach, massage your partner's chest muscles with your fingertips.

- Next, experiment giving your partner a tender scalp massage.

- You can also massage your partner's arms.

- To end, place your hands lightly over your partner's eyes, close your eyes, and rest together.

- Breathe ten or more times in unison.

- Feel how much you love each other.

- Rest deeply together!

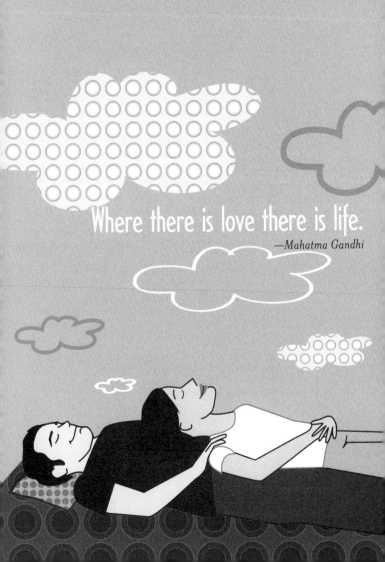

Where there is love there is life.

—*Mahatma Gandhi*

· Mini Romantic Getaway ·
Table for Two

Food is an exotic addition to your Lovers' Massage session.

Mangoes, strawberries, chocolate, honey, ice cream, whipped cream, and bubbly drinks can make wonderful treats.

An intimate way to eat is to feed each other; this should provide lots of fun and laughter.

Ask your partner which food he or she wants, and slowly tempt your partner with a mouthful.

Be patient, and try not to cheat and feed yourself!

It will be an amusing and intimate meal together.

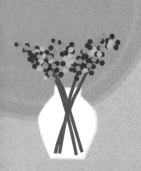

If you want to be loved, be lovable.

—*Ovid*

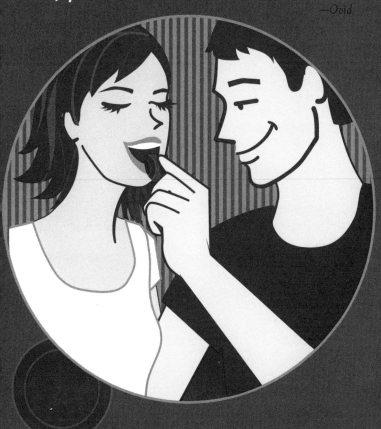

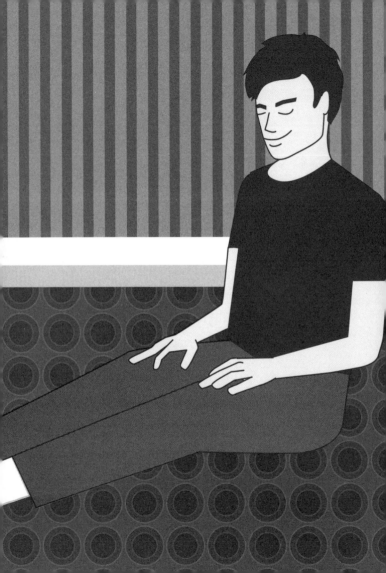

PART 3:
Reconnecting Partner Massage
Soothing Sitting–Up Series

This massage series will stimulate
the energy flow between the hips
and the head and is very relaxing.

Necking
Love Taps

- Your partner sits up into a forward bend.
- Kneel behind him.
- Rub his neck and shoulders with your hands.
- With loose fists, gently tap the muscles across his shoulders and between his shoulder blades.
- Chop in a slow, steady rhythm of love.
- Take five deep breaths together, and remind him to let his shoulders drop.

Neck Squeeze

- Tilt his head forward.
- Interlace your fingers, and gently squeeze together the heels of your palms up and down his neck.
- Try squeezing his neck and hold for a deep breath.
- Ask him how the pressure feels and repeat.

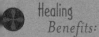

Healing Benefits: *Helps relieve headaches and neck and shoulder tension.*

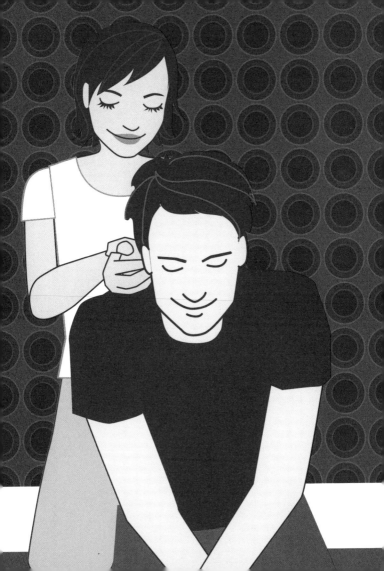

Neck Stretch

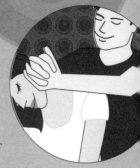

- Rest your left forearm on her left shoulder.

- Carefully position your right forearm against the left side of her head just above her ear.

- Slowly and very slightly press both your forearms in opposite directions.

- Take great care not to overstretch her neck.

- Ask her how the pressure feels, and hold for a count of ten.

Repeat this series on the other side.

Helping Hug

- Wrap her arms in opposite directions as if she were giving herself a hug.

- Next, wrap your arms around her, with your hands on her opposite elbows.

- Have her lean back against your chest, and lovingly support her.

- Pull her elbows, and ask her how the stretch feels.

- Relax, and take five deep, calming breaths together.

- This is a good time for sweet kisses on the back of her neck.

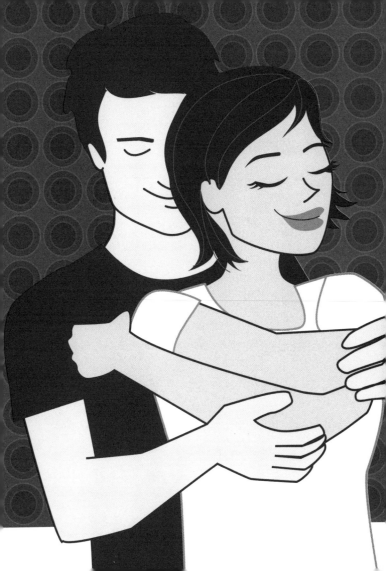

Open Up!

Arm in Arm Together

- Your partner sits up into a forward bend.
- Kneel behind him.
- Interlace his hands behind his head.
- Wrap your arms under his, and clasp your hands over the top of his hands.
- Gently stretch his head forward for a nice neck stretch.
- Ask him how the stretch feels, and hold for a count of ten.

Heart Opening

- Keep his hands interlaced behind his head.
- Slide your arms under his armpits.
- Brace your forearms against his arms.
- Push your upper body gently against his back.
- Stretch his arms back with your hands or forearms.
- Ask him how this stretch feels, and hold for a count of ten.

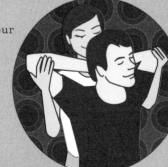

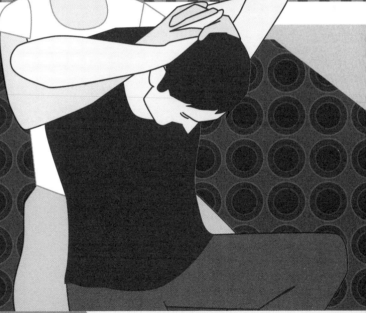

We find rest in those we love, and we provide a resting place in ourselves for those who love us.

—*Saint Bernard of Clairvaux*

Healing Benefits: *Improves spinal flexibility and relieves shoulder tension.*

Head over Heels
Friendly Forward Bend

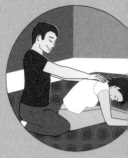

- Your partner sits up into a forward bend.

- Sit up behind her, and push on her back slowly forward.

- Reach around and squeeze with your fingers and thumbs the muscles in between her neck and shoulders.

- With your thumbs, knuckles, and palms, massage up and down on either side of her spine.

- Make loose fists, and gently pound the muscles along her spine.

- To end, gently lean forward onto her back and rest, taking several deep breaths together.

- Feel the intimate relaxation and remember to breathe deeply.

Buddy Back Bend

- Sit about two to three feet behind her.

- Reach around her, and grab her wrists.

- Lean back, drawing her arms behind her.

- Place your feet against her back on either side of her spine, just below her shoulder blades.

- Pull on her arms, and press with your feet to create a strong backward shoulder stretch.

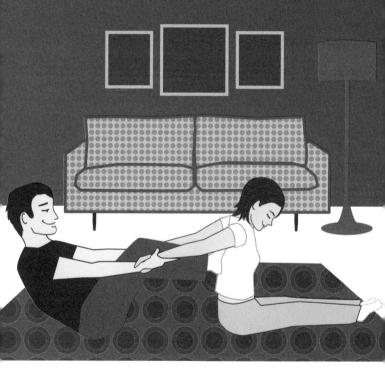

Love me when I least deserve it,
because that's when I really need it.

—Swedish proverb

Healing
Benefits: *Improves spinal flexibility
and eases stiffness in the back.*

Fabulous Five Massages

"Heeling" Massage

- The receiver sits up into a forward bend.
- Sit about three feet behind the receiver.
- Lie down, and rest your feet on the receiver's upper back.
- Press and walk your heels up and down the receiver's back.
- Dig your heels into the sore spots between the receiver's spine and shoulder blades.
- Rest your heels on top of the receiver's shoulders, and push downward.
- With caution, lift your pelvis up into the air for extra leverage.
- Ask the receiver how he or she likes the pressure.
- This is a heavenly way to give a back massage without lifting a finger!
- Take ten long, deep breaths together.

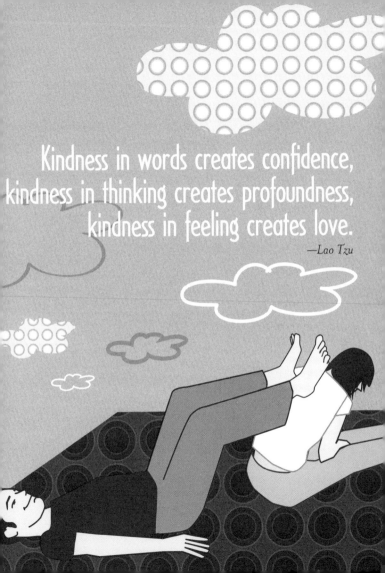

Kindness in words creates confidence,
kindness in thinking creates profoundness,
kindness in feeling creates love.

—*Lao Tzu*

Mini Romantic Getaway
Two to Tango

- Play your favorite dance music.
- Dance together! Let go! Open up!
- Move your hips to the rhythm of the beat.
- Let go, and have fun dancing.
- Enjoy the playful interaction with your partner.
- Take turns leading and following each other's dance steps.
- When you are ready to slow things down, play a love song.
- Wrap your arms around your partner.
- Take turns hugging and squeezing each other tightly.
- Hold on tight to your partner, and massage each other.
- Let yourself melt into your partner's embrace while you rub each other's backs.

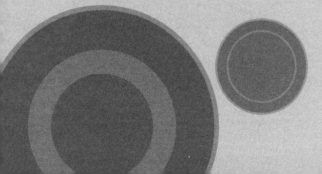

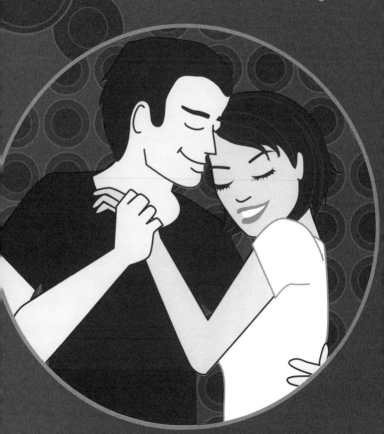

Love is the beauty of the soul.

—Saint Augustine

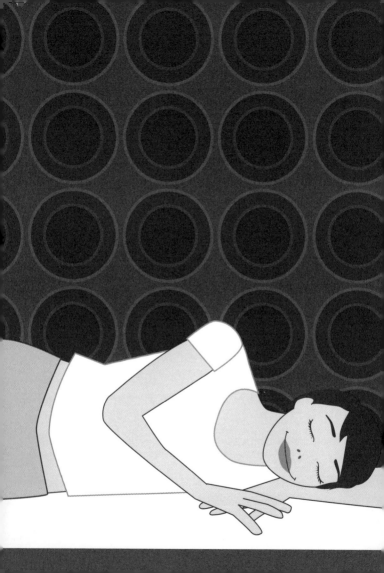

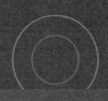

PART 4:
Reviving Partner Massage
Supportive Side Series

This massage series will stimulate the energy flow on the sides of the body and has a calming effect on the nervous system.

Sideways Samba
One Step

- Your partner lies on his right side, with his feet two feet apart.

- Sit with your legs out in front and in-between his legs.

- Grasp both of his ankles for leverage, and use your left foot to press up and down on the back side of his left thigh.

- Generate pressure by leaning back and pulling both his ankles with your hands.

- Ask him how he likes the pressure.

Two Step

- Tuck your left foot behind his left knee, and cross his left foot over your left shin.

- Tuck his toes in behind your knee, holding his heel with your left hand.

- Press up and down his thigh and buttocks using your right foot.

- This feels great on the buttocks!

- Breathe, relax together, and have some fun.

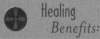

Healing Benefits: *Eases hip and sciatic pain and relaxes hamstrings.*

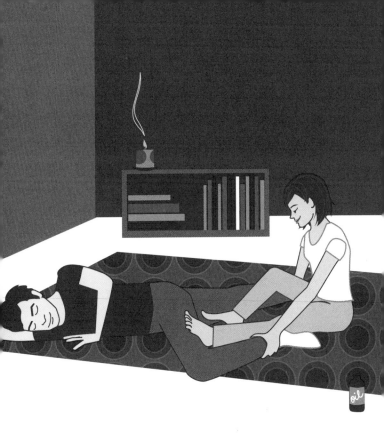

If you are patient in one moment
of anger, you will escape a hundred
days of sorrow.

—*Chinese proverb*

Got Your Back!
Push Back

- Your partner lies on her right side.

- Kneel behind her back.

- Make sure her left leg is bent so her body won't tip over.

- Rub your palm along the left side of her spine in a rocking motion.

- Use your forearm and elbow to massage her left hip and buttock.

Shoulder Circles

- Kneel behind your partner's midsection.

- Slide one arm under her left arm, interlace your fingers, and firmly grasp her shoulder between your hands.

- Slowly rotate her left shoulder in wide circles in both directions.

- Don't work too hard; use your body weight for leverage.

Healing Benefits: *Restores shoulder mobility and relieves upper-back tension.*

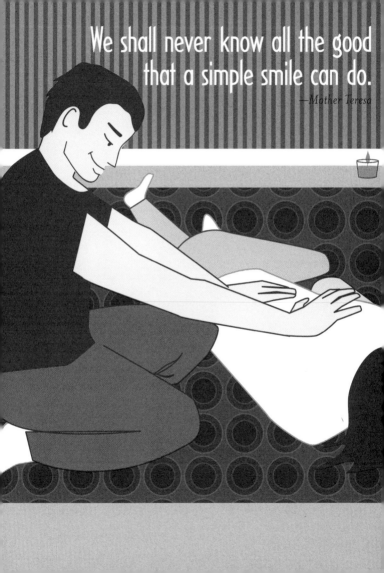

We shall never know all the good that a simple smile can do.
—*Mother Teresa*

Helping Hand

Arm Squeeze

- Your partner lies on his right side.

- Kneel behind his back.

- Stretch his left arm back, and rest it on your lap.

- Rhythmically squeeze, with both your hands, up and down his arm.

Have him roll over, and repeat this series on the other side of his body.

Hand Squeeze

- With both of your hands, massage his left hand, squeezing his palm and fingers.

- Lean back, and pull his left hand to stretch out his arm.

- Next, using your index finger and thumb, squeeze up and down each of his fingers (a little oil or lotion will help).

- Pull each finger separately, using a firm, sliding stroke.

- Breathe and relax together!

- Take your time, and nurture his hardworking hands.

Have him roll over, and repeat this series on the other side of his body.

Healing
Benefits: *Relieves stiffness in the arms, wrists, and hands.*

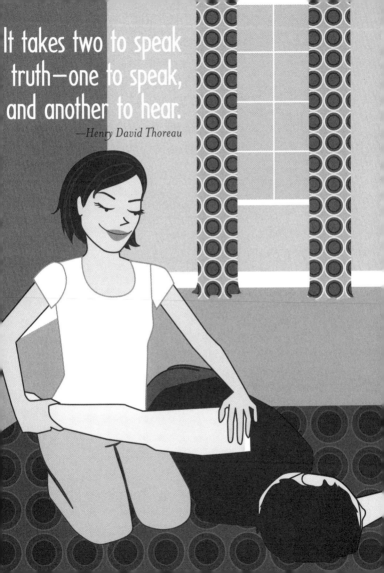

Fabulous Five Massages

Spooning Savasana

Lie down together on your sides, one behind the other in the spooning position.

Cuddle with your partner, and lie motionless.

Breathe in unison ten or more times.

Your bodies will naturally connect together.

Your love and care for your partner will grow with each breath.

Next, the partner behind can lean back and massage the other's upper back and shoulders.

Rub the muscles between the shoulder blade and spine on each side.

Both partners can roll over and reverse the process.

Cuddling is a great way for both of you to relax and be intimate!

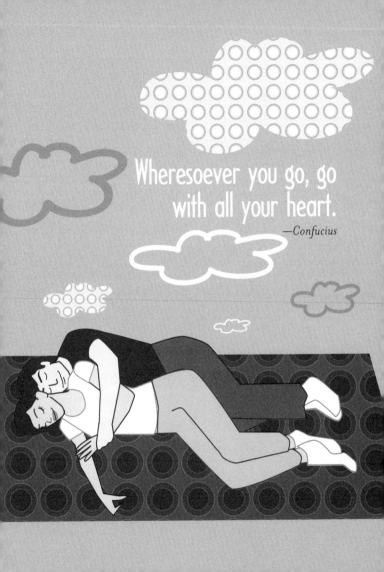

Wheresoever you go, go
with all your heart.
—*Confucius*

Mini Romantic Getaway
Sharing Circle

..... Take turns talking to each other.

..... One person listens while the other speaks.

..... Debrief your busy day.

..... Let go of your stresses and worries.

..... Simply relax and be with each other.

..... Give each other space to speak freely without interruption.

..... Next, spend time telling your partner all the things you love about him or her.

..... Acknowledgments help partners feel connected.

..... Practice being a good listener.

..... Speak honestly, and listen with all your attention.

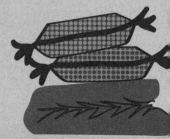

Kind words can be short and easy to speak, but their echoes are truly endless.

—*Mother Teresa*

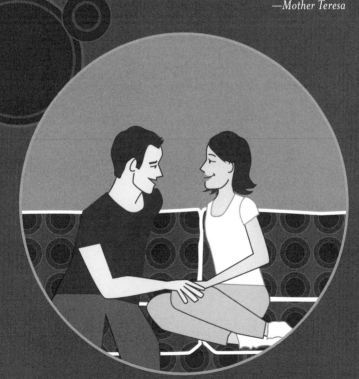

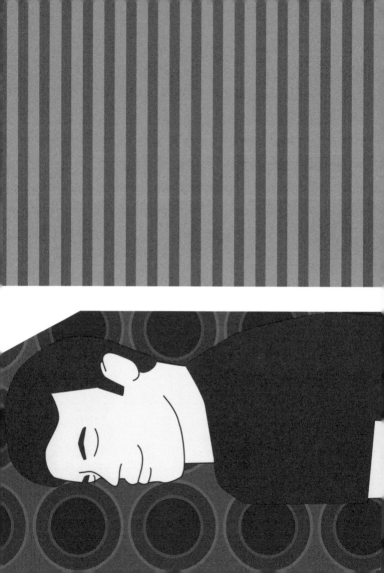

PART 5:
Romantic Partner Massage
Sensual Full–Body Series

This massage series will stimulate the
energy flow in the entire body and
is very energizing and relaxing.

Sole to Sole

This is a deep foot massage, so be careful.

- Your partner lies facedown.

- Place a pillow or folded blanket under his feet and ankles to create adequate padding.

- Stand by his feet, facing away from him, and walk your heels on his feet.

- Ask him how the pressure feels.

- Carefully and gently rock back and forth, pressing your heels into the soles of his feet.

- Balance your weight using your toes, and lean slightly backward to apply deeper pressure.

- Take five deep breaths, and then step off.

If he loves a deep foot massage, he will love this technique:

You can also try using your knees rather than your feet on his soles.

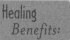

Healing Benefits: *Increases flexibility and circulation in the feet and creates deep relaxation.*

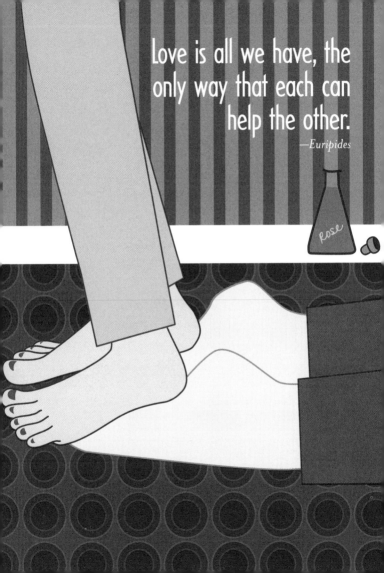

Baby Got Back!
Leg Press

- Your partner lies facedown, with her feet two feet apart.

- Kneel between her legs.

- Use your thumbs to squeeze the soles of her feet and the inside of her legs.

- Rub the buttocks with loose fists.

- Rock forward and back to create a calm, rhythmic motion to help her relax.

- Remind her to take long, deep breaths.

Back Press

- Slide your body up closer to her back.

- Press with your palms on either side of her spine, fingers directed outward.

- Use both hands to apply pressure slowly up and down the back.

- Keep your arms straight so you can use your body weight for leverage.

- Have her exhale deeply each time you press downward.

- Next, gently caress her whole back, using your fingertips like feathers.

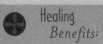

Healing Benefits: *Stimulates energy flow through the legs and back and calms the nervous system.*

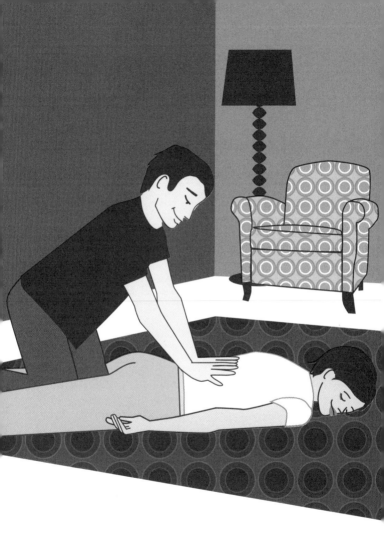

Romantic Rub
Palm Connection

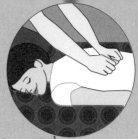

- Your partner lies facedown.

- Kneel above her head.

- Rub your hands together quickly to create heat.

- Rest your hands on her upper back, and tune in to her breathing.

- Next, rock your palms along her spine all the way down to her buttocks.

- Use your knuckles to rub in-between the spine and shoulder blades.

- Repeat these strokes several times.

Thumb Circles

- Use your thumbs to massage each side of her spine.

- Rest your hands on her back to help balance your thumb movements.

- Move both thumbs in small circular motions.

- Slide up and down the spine several times.

- Next, place both of your thumbs on one side of the spine between the shoulder blade and the spine.

- Use both thumbs to massage around one shoulder blade, and then switch.

- Make small circles with your thumbs in an alternating movement.

- Remind her to relax and enjoy the soothing back relief.

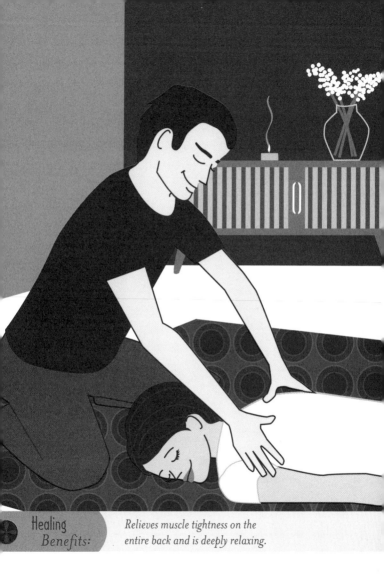

Healing Benefits: *Relieves muscle tightness on the entire back and is deeply relaxing.*

Full Body Bliss
Hand Circles

- Your partner lies facedown.
- Kneel beside her near her buttocks.
- Gently touch the palms of your hands on the back side of her body.
- Let your hands travel spontaneously up and down, from head to toe.
- Make circling hand movements and experiment with the depth of pressure.
- Try making your touch as light as a feather.

Forearm Free Flow

- Rest both of your forearms on her back.
- Use your own body weight as leverage.
- Massage with your forearms along the muscles; try to avoid the bony areas.
- Travel in a smooth motion around her body.
- When she moans happily, it's good to stop and apply pressure on the area she likes.
- Ask her if she wants more or less pressure.

Healing
Benefits: *Helps loosen the body joints and provides profound relaxation.*

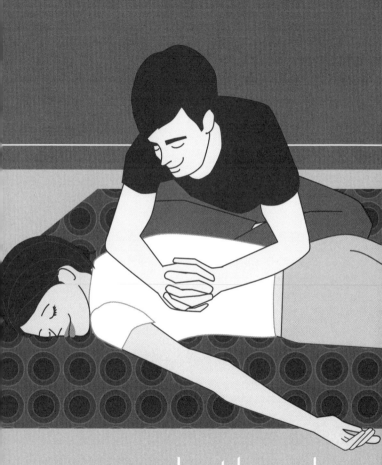

love takes up where
knowledge leaves off.
—Saint Thomas Aquinas

Love Seat

··········
*Be careful when giving these two techniques
if you are a lot heavier than your partner.*

Sitting Forward

- Your partner lies facedown.

- Sit on his buttocks, kneeling your legs on each side of his body.

- Ask him if your body weight feels good to him.

- Place both your hands on his back.

- Use your palms or knuckles to rub his back muscles.

- Work your way up and down along his spine.

Resting Bodies

- Gently lower your body weight on top of him, your front to his back.

- Brace your arms and feet on the ground to lighten your weight.

- Ask him if your body weight feels good.

- Take five deep, relaxing breaths, and let your tensions melt away together.

- Using your whole body is very intimate and relaxing for both the giver and receiver.

- Whisper in his ear, "I love you."

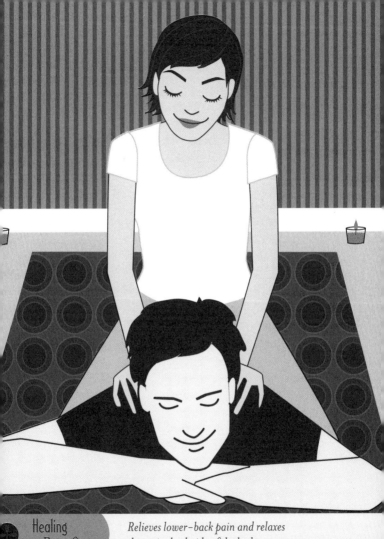

Healing Benefits: *Relieves lower-back pain and relaxes the entire back side of the body.*

Child's Pose for Partners

- Have your partner kneel facedown so his upper body is resting on his knees.

- Kneel behind him, and rest your hands on his back for a few deep breaths together.

- Next, rub the muscles along his spine with your thumbs or knuckles.

- Tap lightly on his back and buttocks with loose fists.

- Lie your upper body down on top of his back.

- Ask him if your body weight feels good to him.

- Take five deep breaths, and relax together.

- This is a nice time to express your love and appreciation for your partner.

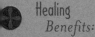

Healing *Benefits:* — *Relieves tension in the lower back and has a nurturing effect.*

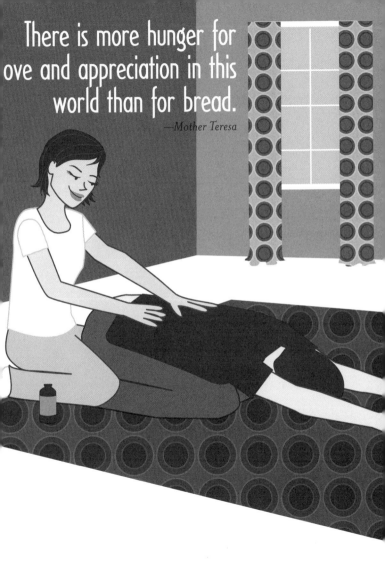

There is more hunger for ove and appreciation in this world than for bread.

—*Mother Teresa*

Fabulous Five Massages

Steamroller Relaxation

• • • Have the receiver lie facedown.

• • • Lower your body over the receiver's body at a right angle.

• • • Slowly roll your body over the receiver like a steamroller. (Carefully around the neck area.)

• • • Repeat from head to toe and back again.

• • • Stop, lie motionless on top of your partner, and feel your body stretch.

• • • Take deep breaths, and experiment rolling your body in different ways.

• • • This is a marvelous way to give your partner quick stress relief.

• • • The heavier partner will need to be careful that his or her weight is not too much.

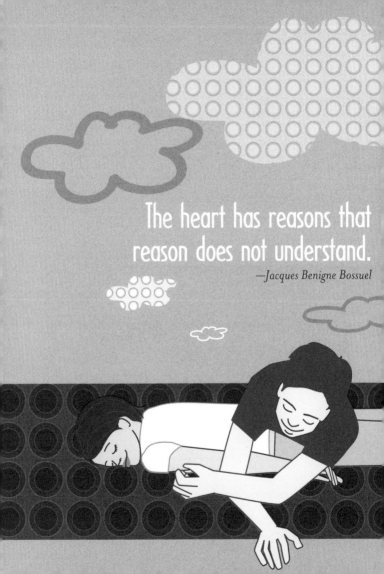

The heart has reasons that
reason does not understand.

—Jacques Benigne Bossuel

Mini Romantic Getaway
Tantric Embrace

- Lie down on your side, face-to-face with your partner.

- Rest your heads on a pillow.

- Comfortably wrap your arms around your partner.

- Take ten long, deep breaths.

- Feel your bodies melting together.

- Gently massage your partner's back.

- Knead your fingers and knuckles into the muscles of the other's upper back between the spine and shoulder blades.

- Give each other a neck rub and scalp massage.

- Feel the connection and deep relaxation that unfolds.

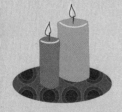

Life without love is like a tree without blossoms or fruit.

—Kahlil Gibran

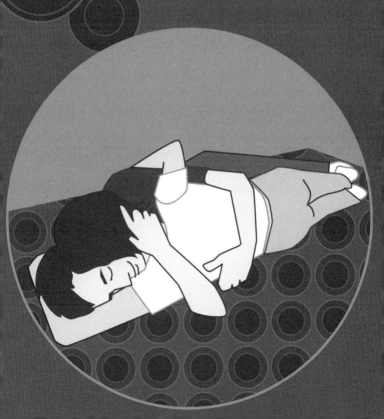

Seduction of the Senses

Use sensual items to tantalize your partner. Try an intoxicating scent, the chilly sensation of an ice cube, or a feather's touch!

Scent of a Rose

Choose a flower that has a nice scent, one you know your partner likes. Caress the flower under the other's nose, allowing him or her to inhale the scent. Slowly run the flower over the entire body. Or try a flower-scented massage oil, such as lavender, geranium, neroli er (orange blossom), jasmine, or ylang-ylang. Use natural water-based massage-oil products that won't stain clothes or bedding.

Cold as Ice

Place an ice cube gently at the top of your partner's spine. Allow it to slowly slide down your partner's back, tingling the spine with its cold sensation. Keep the ice cube moving!

Light as a Feather

Feathers are wonderfully sensual when brushed across the skin. Use a soft feather to caress your partner's body, slowly tickling and teasing his or her skin. Tickle the toes and feet to make your partner giggle.

Acknowledgments

A special thanks to Daisy Talleur for her incredible support. Also, a special thanks to John Mapleback, Lisa Campbell, Tana Martin, Alison St. John, Damien Inglis, Jodi Davis, and Yosel Tarnofsky for taking good care of me! And thanks to all of my Lovers' Massage buddies!

Biography

Darrin Zeer teaches Lovers' Yoga & Massage Retreats at resorts and yoga studios around the world. He also teaches Office Yoga to corporations all over America.

Darrin spent seven years traveling and studying yoga and massage throughout Asia. He has appeared on CNN, in the *Yoga Journal*, *Time* magazine, and the *New York Times*. Darrin is also the author of *Lovers' Yoga*, *Office Yoga*, *Office Spa*, *Office Feng Shui*, *Everyday Calm*, *Travel Yoga*, and the Office Stress Emergency Kit (all from Chronicle Books). He has given more than 10,000 massages.

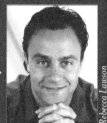

Rebecca Lawson

For more information about Darrin's Lovers' Yoga & Massage Romantic Retreats, go to

www.loversmassage.com.

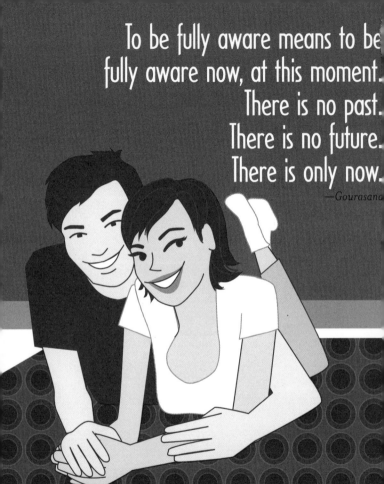

To be fully aware means to be
fully aware now, at this moment.
There is no past.
There is no future.
There is only now.

—*Gourasana*

*Enjoy a relaxing Lovers' Massage
adventure for two!*